# Cambridge Elements ≡

Elements in Emergency Neurosurgery
edited by
Nihal Gurusinghe
*Lancashire Teaching Hospital NHS Trust*
Peter Hutchinson
*University of Cambridge, Society of British Neurological Surgeons and Royal
College of Surgeons of England*
Ioannis Fouyas
*Royal College of Surgeons of Edinburgh*
Naomi Slator
*North Bristol NHS Trust*
Ian Kamaly-Asl
*Royal Manchester Children's Hospital*
Peter Whitfield
*University Hospitals Plymouth NHS Trust*

# SPINAL DISCITIS AND EPIDURAL ABSCESS

Damjan Veljanoski
*University Hospitals Plymouth NHS Trust and the
University of Plymouth*
Pragnesh Bhatt
*Aberdeen Royal Infirmary and The University
of Aberdeen*

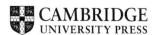

CAMBRIDGE
UNIVERSITY PRESS

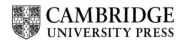

# CAMBRIDGE
## UNIVERSITY PRESS

Shaftesbury Road, Cambridge CB2 8EA, United Kingdom

One Liberty Plaza, 20th Floor, New York, NY 10006, USA

477 Williamstown Road, Port Melbourne, VIC 3207, Australia

314–321, 3rd Floor, Plot 3, Splendor Forum, Jasola District Centre,
New Delhi – 110025, India

103 Penang Road, #05–06/07, Visioncrest Commercial, Singapore 238467

Cambridge University Press is part of Cambridge University Press & Assessment,
a department of the University of Cambridge.

We share the University's mission to contribute to society through the pursuit of
education, learning and research at the highest international levels of excellence.

www.cambridge.org
Information on this title: www.cambridge.org/9781009494823

DOI: 10.1017/9781009409391

© Damjan Veljanoski and Pragnesh Bhatt 2024

First published 2024

*A catalogue record for this publication is available from the British Library.*

ISBN 978-1-009-49482-3 Hardback
ISBN 978-1-009-40940-7 Paperback
ISSN 2755-0656 (online)
ISSN 2755-0648 (print)

# Spinal Discitis and Epidural Abscess

Elements in Emergency Neurosurgery

DOI: 10.1017/9781009409391
First published online: June 2024

Damjan Veljanoski
*University Hospitals Plymouth NHS Trust and the University of Plymouth*

Pragnesh Bhatt
*Aberdeen Royal Infirmary and The University of Aberdeen*

**Author for correspondence:** Damjan Veljanoski, veljanoski@doctors.org.uk

**Abstract:** Spinal infections (SIs) are rare conditions affecting the intervertebral disc, vertebral body, and/or adjacent spinal tissues. The lumbar region is most commonly involved, followed by the thoracic and cervical regions. Patients present with varied, non-specific clinical features leading to diagnostic and treatment delays. Clinicians need to have a low threshold to suspect SI. In this Element, two real-life cases of patients with SIs will be presented first. Core knowledge will be reviewed next, followed by diagnostic pitfalls and clinical pearls. Finally, the 'typical' clinical workflow for a patient with SI will be presented and the various treatment options will be explored.

**Keywords:** spinal infection, spondylodiscitis, spinal epidural abscess, vertebral osteomyelitis, discitis

ISBNs: 9781009494823 (HB), 9781009409407 (PB), 9781009409391 (OC)
ISSNs: 2755-0656 (online), 2755-0648 (print)

# Contents

# 1 Clinical Scenarios

## 1.1 A Patient with Spondylodiscitis Treated Conservatively

A 72-year-old man was admitted to hospital with a three-month history of lumbar back pain radiating to his thighs, with acute worsening over the preceding two weeks and bilateral L5 radicular pain, saddle paraesthesia, and new bladder disturbance. He was bed-bound due to limb weakness and pain.

Over the preceding three-month period, the patient had consulted an osteopath and a physiotherapist, with little relief. There was no precipitating injury. Plain radiographs at that time showed disc space narrowing at L2/3. The patient had also recently been treated in hospital for a urinary tract infection secondary to coagulase-negative *Staphylococcus*.

The patient's past medical history was positive for coronary artery bypass graft and percutaneous coronary intervention, hypothyroidism, hypertension, and previous stroke. C-reactive protein (CRP) was mildly raised but white cell count (WCC) and neutrophils were normal. Blood and urine samples did not yield any organisms on microbiological analysis. A magnetic resonance imaging (MRI) scan of the lumbar spine and sacrum was performed, which demonstrated fluid signal in the L4/5 disc as well as end-plate destruction and bone marrow oedema consistent with L4/5 spondylodiscitis (Figures 1 and 2). There was no significant collection present and no evidence of cauda equina compression.

A decision was made to manage the patient conservatively under the care of the Infectious Disease team. Intravenous ceftriaxone was commenced, completing six weeks of therapy, before switching to oral therapy, for a further 20 weeks.

Following an improvement in his symptoms and CRP, the antibiotics were stopped. However, the back and lower limb pain persisted so the patient was started on neuropathic analgesics, which he responded to well (see Figure 3 for the clinical algorithm summary for this patient).

## 1.2 A Patient with a Spinal Epidural Abscess Treated Surgically

A 39-year-old man presented to hospital with chest pain and loss of sensation in his limbs. He had injured his back following a fall a few weeks previously when he was also treated for alcohol withdrawal and septicaemia. Past medical history included heavy alcohol intake with secondary seizures.

He was found to have chest infection and weakness, affecting his whole left lower limb. Intravenous Tazocin was started to treat the pneumonia, and he required urinary catheterisation.

Overnight, he developed a sensory level at the T4 dermatome and right lower limb weakness. Plain radiographs demonstrated a healing wedge fracture at T7.

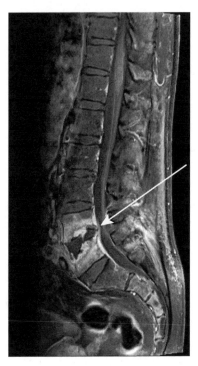

**Figure 1** T1 weighted sagittal MRI with contrast. Red arrow points
to L4/5 spondylodiscitis with destruction of the vertebral endplates and bone
marrow oedema.

An MRI scan showed a spinal epidural abscess (SEA; see Figures 4 and 5). He
underwent T2-4 laminectomy and drainage of the SEA.

The patient received a four-month course of antibiotic therapy; however, he
re-presented with *Staphylococcus aureus* bacteraemia and worsening radiological appearances, including a kyphotic deformity. Due to this complex
kyphotic deformity, the patient underwent elective transthoracic spinal stabil-
isation (see Figure 6 for the clinical algorithm summary for this patient).

## 2 Definitions

### 2.1 Discitis

An infection of the intervertebral disc only.

### 2.2 Spondylodiscitis

An infection of the intervertebral disc and the vertebral body. Also known as
vertebral osteomyelitis.

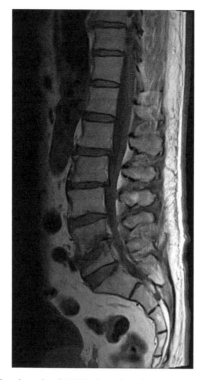

**Figure 2** T1 weighted sagittal MRI showing the post-treatment appearances of the L4/5 spondylodiscitis.

## 2.3 Spinal Abscess

This can be classified anatomically in relation to the spinal cord and dura: epidural (rare conditions, associated with high mortality), subdural, and intramedullary (extremely rare and usually due to an underlying spinal cord pathology).

## 2.4 Paraspinal Abscess

This affects paraspinal tissues, most commonly the iliopsoas muscle.

## 3 Core Knowledge

### 3.1 Epidemiology

Spinal infections account for 2–7% of all musculoskeletal infections [1]. In a review of 669 patients aged greater than 55 who presented to their general practice with back pain, it was found that none had spinal infection [2]. Furthermore, it has been estimated that the point prevalence of infection in patients with non-mechanical lower back pain is 0.01% in primary care [3] and

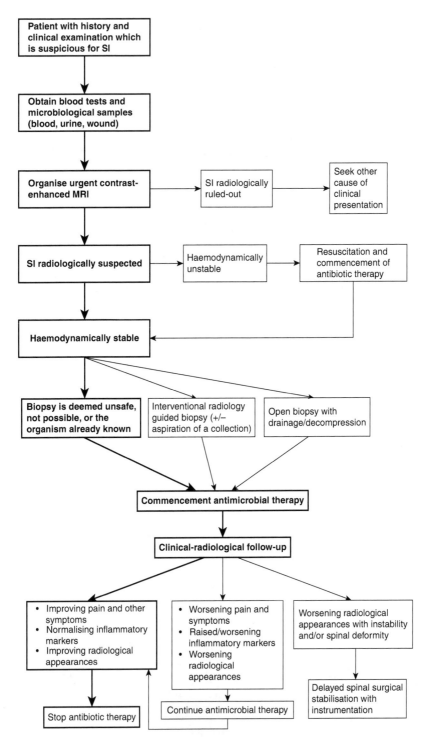

**Figure 3** Clinical algorithm for case 1.

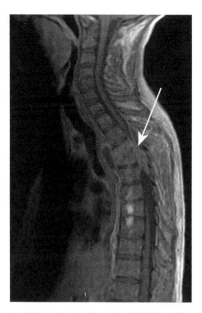

**Figure 4** Preoperative T1 weighted sagittal MRI with contrast. Red arrow points to a SEA at the level of T4.

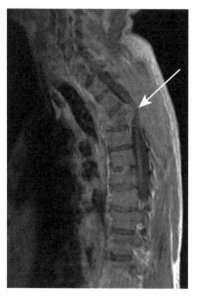

**Figure 5** Post-operative T1 weighted sagittal MRI with contrast. Red arrow points to kyphosis of the thoracic spine at the level of the SEA.

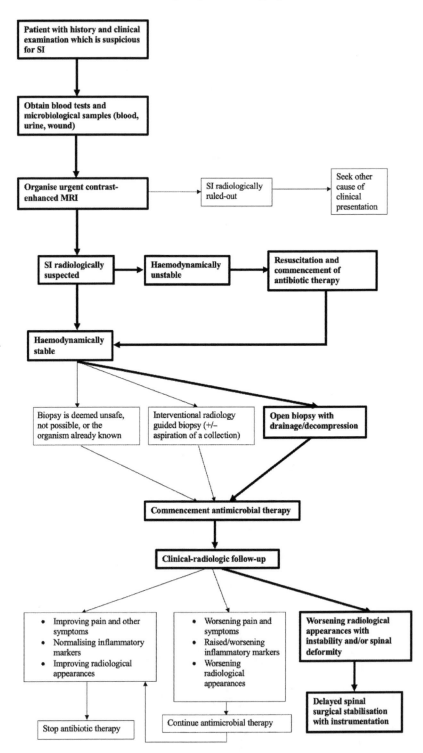

**Figure 6** Clinical algorithm for case 2.

1.2% in a tertiary setting [4]. There is a bimodal distribution with one group below 20 years of age and another within the 50–70 years of age group. Males are affected more frequently than females with ratios ranging from 2:1 to 5:1 [5–7]. An increase in the incidence of SIs in recent decades has been noted [8]. This could be due to improvements in diagnostic pathways and imaging techniques, an ageing population with more comorbidities, increasing intravenous drug use (IVDU), and more frequent spinal operations [9, 6].

## 3.2 Classification

Spinal infections can be pyogenic or non-pyogenic, depending on the underlying disease process and causative organisms. Pyogenic SIs tend to result in purulence and a marked neutrophilic response due to infection with bacteria, or less commonly, parasites or fungi, whereas non-pyogenic SIs are characterised by a granulomatous response. Granulomatous SIs are characterised by formation of a granuloma, which is a collection of macrophages, matrix, and inflammatory cells [10]. Granulomatous infections can be classified as typical and atypical, according to the causative bacterium, fungus, or parasite. *Mycobacterium tuberculosis* (also known as Pott's disease) is a typical pathogen, and accounts for the majority of granulomatous SIs. Atypical organisms include the likes of *Brucella*, *Actinomyces*, and *Nocardia* [10]. Granulomatous SIs will be dealt with separately, in Element 84 (Shetty, Bhatt, *Cranial and Spinal Tuberculosis Infections including Acute Presentations*, Elements in Emergency Neurosurgery, Cambridge University Press, forthcoming). Spinal infections can also be described anatomically, in relation to the spinal cord, spinal canal, dura, and paraspinal muscles. They can be spontaneous or iatrogenic.

## 3.3 Anatomy

A spinal segment consists of two vertebral bodies separated by one intervertebral disc. A cadaveric study of the vertebral arterial and venous blood supply has revealed the detailed vascular anatomy of the spinal column [11]. The vertebral arterial supply originates from nutrient vessels, and their structure is similar across the cervical, thoracic, and lumbar regions. A vertebral, intercostal, or lumbar segmental artery lying in close proximity to each vertebral body gives off smaller vessels which penetrate the cortex and supply the marrow centrally. Furthermore, there is a posterior spinal artery branch in the intervertebral foramen which divides into ascending and descending branches that also anastomose with the superior and inferior segments, and from the contralateral side. Thus, an anastomotic network exists on the dorsal surface of each vertebral body. From this network originate three to four nutrient arteries which enter the vertebral body via its dorsal surface via a large, central foramen. The segmental arteries and the smaller posterior spinal arterioles anastomose freely.

Conversely, the venous drainage of the vertebral body has been described as tree-like when viewed in the coronal plane [11]. Within the vertebral body form tiny tributaries which meet centrally and collect into a large, valveless channel that exits the vertebral body via the dorsal, centrally located nutrient foramen. These vessels drain into an expansive plexus that lines the vertebral canal. There are further, irregular connections between the tributaries of the vertebral body and the veins on the ventral and lateral surfaces of the vertebral bodies. Batson's vertebral plexus describes the aforementioned spinal and paraspinal venous plexus.

This cadaveric study with injection of vessels found that spread of disease processes to the vertebral bone marrow occurred more freely via the nutrient arteries and less freely via the less accessible paravertebral venous system [11].

In childhood, the blood supply to the intervertebral disc originates from small perforating vessels. However, in adulthood, these blood vessels degrade, and the intervertebral disc becomes virtually avascular and hence more likely to get infected. In spondylodiscitis, adjacent spinal segments can be affected.

## 3.4 Pathophysiology

Spinal infections can arise due to haematogenous or contiguous spread of, or direct contamination with, infecting microorganisms [12]. Haematogenous spread is most common and two theories involving the arterial and venous systems exist [13].

Arterial spread is thought to occur when a systemic infection or bacteraemia generates septic emboli that deposit in the small metaphyseal arteries of the vertebral endplates resulting in an area of infarction [11]. A localised infection develops, which spreads through the vertebral body and into the adjacent intervertebral disc, which is poorly vascularised. Spinal abscesses and paraspinal collections develop when this infection spreads beyond the margins of the spinal column.

Venous spread is believed to be less commonly implicated in SIs [11]. This may occur when intra-abdominal or pelvic sources of infection spread via the venous, valveless Batson's plexus draining the spinal column [14]. Contiguous spread occurs when there is spread of infection from a local area. An iatrogenic cause is direct inoculation, which occurs most commonly following a spinal operation, spinal/epidural injection, and lumbar puncture [15]. Spinal epidural abscess (SEA) can occur as a complication of insertion of epidural catheters for anaesthesia [16].

## 3.5 Clinical Presentation

The presenting symptoms of SIs are generally non-specific and develop insidiously. There can be a significant delay between the onset of symptoms and the diagnosis of SI. Patients most commonly report neck or back pain which is non-mechanical, constant, and not relieved by rest [17]. The pain is usually worse at night and can awaken the patient [18]. Neurological symptoms include limb weakness, altered sensation, altered mobility, and disturbance of urinary or bowel function (depending on the spinal level involved) [19]. Neurological deficits are usually a late feature of spondylodiscitis when there is severe disc destruction and vertebral collapse. However, in the case of spinal epidural abscess, there is earlier neural compression and compromise. Other features include fever, chills, rigors, weight loss, and fatigue.

## 3.6 Risk Factors

Risk factors for SI can be classified as those which increase the susceptibility to infection and those which directly cause infection. Predisposing conditions include diabetes mellitus, immunosuppression, malignancy, alcohol excess, rheumatoid arthritis, spinal fracture or trauma, chronic kidney disease, acute or chronic infection, and immobility. Risk factors that may directly cause infection include recent spinal procedures, spinal trauma, or fracture, IVDU, and implantable devices or foreign bodies.

## 3.7 Causative Microbiological Organisms

*Staphylococcus aureus* (including methicillin-resistant *Staphylococcus aureus*) is the most common causative organism of SIs. Coagulase-negative staphylococci, *Escherichia coli*, and *Proteus* species are frequently isolated as well, and the latter two are more common in patients with a urinary tract infection. Gram-negative organisms, such as *Klebsiella* and *Pseudomonas*, should be considered in patients with a history of IVDU. *Mycobacterium tuberculosis* and fungi, such as *Aspergillus* species, *Candida* species, and *Cryptococcus neoformans*, are rarer and these are seen in immunocompromised hosts.

# 4 Typical Clinical Pathways and Any Possible Variations

## 4.1 Full History and Examination

Elicit symptoms are suggestive of SI and identify risk factors, relevant comorbidities, recent infections, or invasive procedures (see Figure 7).

Perform a full neurological examination and a systemic search for wounds and ulcers. Check for incisional scars suggesting prior surgery. Check for point

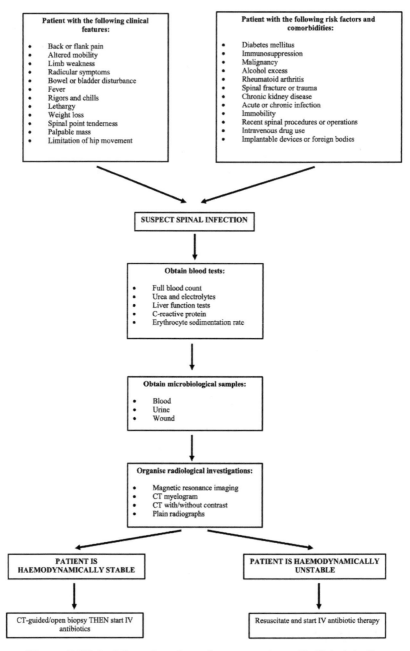

**Figure 7** Clinical flow chart for patient presenting with SI (original).

tenderness along the spinal column and paravertebral muscle spasm. Assess the patient's spinal alignment noting any kyphosis or scoliosis.

Look for fever, tachycardia, and signs of sepsis.

## 4.2 Infection Screen

Send blood tests to include a full blood count (FBC) with a differential white cell count, urea and electrolytes, liver function tests, and CRP, as a direct measure of acute inflammation. In some countries, erythrocyte sedimentation rate is performed, which is an alternative, indirect measure of inflammation, but this is less sensitive than CRP to the acute phase response. Admission CRP levels and WCC are prognostic markers for the likelihood of isolating a causative microorganism from cultures obtained from either blood or biopsy samples [20].

## 4.3 Indications for Admission to Neurosurgery

Neurosurgical wards provide specialist nursing and multidisciplinary care to patients with neurological deficits (e.g., specialist spinal care). Patients with established or worsening neurological deficits, worsening pain, spinal instability, evidence of spinal cord or cauda equina compression on imaging, post-operative SI, and/or systemic illness warrant review by a neurosurgeon to organise expedient imaging and treatment. Close team working with and input from the microbiology team is essential to optimising the patient's antimicrobial therapy and treatment course.

## 4.4 Microbiological Investigations

Send blood cultures from at least two peripheral venous sites to maximise the likelihood of isolating a causative organism. Obtain a sample of urine as infection of the urinary tract is a common source of sepsis and SI. Send wound swabs for microscopy, culture, and sensitivity.

## 4.5 Imaging

### 4.5.1 General

Order a plain chest radiograph to rule out a pulmonary infective focus and as a preoperative work-up for patients with cardiorespiratory comorbidities. Perform a post-void residual bladder scan in patients complaining of urinary difficulties to rule out urinary retention secondary to cauda equina compression.

### 4.5.2 Magnetic Resonance Imaging

The advantages of contrast (gadolinium)-enhanced MRI include excellent resolution of soft tissues and the lack of ionising radiation. Magnetic resonance imaging is contra-indicated in patients with ferro-metallic foreign bodies such as implantable cardiac pacemakers and defibrillators (modern devices can be disabled for MRI in liaison with cardiology), some neurostimulation devices, cochlear implants, and implantable drug infusion devices. Magnetic resonance imaging may be unsuitable for patients with a large body habitus or severe claustrophobia. Early MRI may not show any abnormalities or only show changes related to chronic degeneration. Typical MRI features of SI are detailed in text box 1. The clinical history should be considered carefully alongside the MRI findings to differentiate infection from neoplasia. Where there is significant uncertainty, FDG positron emission tomography combined with computerised tomography (CT) imaging or Gallium citrate scintigraphy, may be pursued. Degenerative (Modic 1) changes should be differentiated from infectious odema (see text box 1).

If early MRI is negative, but suspicion for SI persists, a repeat MRI with contrast after one to three weeks should be performed [21]. For patients with lower back pain and a normal lumbo-sacral MRI scan, a whole-spine MRI is required to rule out occult lesions causing referred pain.

### 4.5.3 CT Myelogram

A CT myelogram is used when MRI is contraindicated. It is performed by injecting a contrast medium into the thecal sac followed by fluoroscopic radiographs and a CT scan.

### 4.5.4 CT with/without IV Contrast

A CT scan provides detail about bony features which aids in assessing the extent of bone involvement as well as to delineate preoperative anatomy for patients undergoing spinal surgery with instrumentation.

### 4.5.5 Plain Radiographs of the Spine

Plain radiographs of the spine have limited utility in diagnosing SI in the acute phase. However, with advancing disease, they may reveal vertebral collapse, end-plate changes, or loss of the intervertebral disc height. Taken at baseline, they may serve as a useful comparison in the future should the patient develop spinal kyphosis or instability. In the latter scenario, flexion-extension radiographs are useful for assessing instability.

## 4.6 Biopsy

A tissue biopsy can be obtained by percutaneous aspiration under CT-guidance or during an open procedure. The decision to undertake a biopsy and its

TEXT BOX 1 MRI FEATURES OF SI [22] [23] [24]

**MRI features of SI**

Vertebral body and/or intervertebral disc:

- ○ T1W: Low signal intensity indicating the presence of fluid within the vertebral body.
- ○ T1W with contrast: Heterogenous contrast enhancement suggesting acute or subacute inflammation. A peripherally enhancing collection may be suggestive of abscess formation.
- ○ T2W: High signal intensity (and further assessed via fat-suppressed T2/STIR sequences).
- ○ DWI and ADC: In pyogenic spondylodiscitis, there is diffusion restriction (high signal on DWI and low signal on the corresponding ADC map).

- • Vertebral endplate destruction
- • Psoas sign: High signal intensity of iliopsoas muscle on T2W imaging (a sign seen in early spondylodiscitis)
- • Modic 1 changes can mimic infection:

  - ○ Modic 1 changes occur acutely in the subchondral surfaces of two adjacent vertebrae as a result of degenerative disease of the intervertebral disc. Appear as low signal on T1, and high signal on T2 or STIR.
  - ○ Differentiating Modic 1 changes from infection; in Modic 1:

    - ▪ There is no abnormal disc signal (hyperintensity) on T2W.
    - ▪ Endplate contours are irregular and intact (whereas they are blurred in infection).
    - ▪ Mixed pattern of inflammation and fat in the oedematous areas of the vertebral body on T1W (whereas there is mainly inflammation in infection).

- • Signs of resolving infection:

  - ○ Normalisation of T1W signal in a vertebral body suggests reconstitution of fatty bone marrow.
  - ○ Decrease in T2W signal in the vertebral body implies sclerosis or fibrosis as part of the healing process.

timing should be considered on a case-by-case basis. It is advantageous to obtain an early biopsy sample as this can increase the likelihood of identifying a causative organism for the SI and help direct antimicrobial therapy according to the sensitivities and susceptibilities of the organism(s). However, it is prudent to delay obtaining a biopsy if the patient is haemodynamically unstable, in which case general resuscitative measures and commencement of intravenous broad-spectrum antibiotics should be prioritised (Figure 7). Commencing antimicrobial therapy prior to undertaking biopsy does not appear to influence the likelihood of isolating an organism later on [25].

## 4.7 Antimicrobial Therapy

The principles underpinning treatment of SI include resuscitation of the haemodynamically unstable patient, control of the infection, and eradication of the source. In almost all cases, a course of antibiotic therapy is required. Several factors should be considered when deciding on the type, duration, and route of antibiotic therapy:

- The antibiotic(s) should cover gram-positive and gram-negative microorganisms, have good penetrance into the central nervous system, be tolerated with a low side-effect profile, and be rationalised once the causative organism is isolated.
- Intravenous antibiotics are usually started, and if suitable, outpatient parenteral antibiotic therapy (OPAT) can be continued. This may necessitate the insertion of a long intravenous line.
- A duration of 6–12 weeks is common, and the decision to switch from OPAT to oral delivery as well as the decision to stop treatment depends on ongoing clinical improvement, satisfactory follow-up imaging, and normalising inflammatory markers.

## 5 Diagnostic Pitfalls and Clinical Pearls

### 5.1 Differential Diagnoses

The most important differential diagnoses for destructive lesions of the spine include infection and neoplasia. Other differential diagnoses include chronic renal failure, ankylosing spondylodiscitis, conditions causing posterior scalloping of the vertebral body (acromegaly, achondroplasia, Marfan syndrome, mucopolysaccharidosis, Ehlers-Danlos syndrome, neurofibromatosis, and dural ectasia), and conditions causing anterior scalloping of the vertebral body (aortic aneurysm, lymphoma, and spinal tuberculosis) [26].

## 5.2 Antibiotic Therapy

Broad-spectrum intravenous antibiotics to cover gram-positive and gram-negative microorganisms should be started. Antibiotic therapy should be rationalised once the infecting organism is isolated or suspected. Follow one's own institutional antimicrobial guidance, which accounts for the prevalence of resistant strains, for example Methicillin-resistant *Staphylococcus aureus*, for which alternative antibiotics, such as Vancomycin, may be required.

## 5.3 Juvenile Spondylodiscitis

Juvenile spondylodiscitis is rare. The condition is difficult to diagnose due to its insidious nature, the non-specific presentation, and the difficulty in obtaining a history and examination from the paediatric patient [27]. This leads to delays in diagnosis and treatment. Presenting clinical features include not wanting to walk or sit, fever, irritability, limping, and back or hip pain [27,28]. In one series, the WCC and CRP levels were normal in 59% and 42% of patients, respectively. Additionally, the blood cultures were positive in 8% of patients and cultures of biopsy or aspirate were positive in 40% [29]. Surgery is indicated when there is vertebral instability and neurological deficit; however, this can be avoided if the infection is treated early and aggressively with antibiotics, often leading to favourable outcomes [27]

## 5.4 Iliopsoas Abscess

An iliopsoas abscess is an infective collection in the retroperitoneal space. It is a rare condition, with an incidence of 0.4 cases for 100,000 people per year [30]. The initial clinical presenting features can be insidious and non-specific, including fever, malaise, and weight loss, as well as abdominal or flank pain, limp, flexion of the ipsilateral hip, lower extremity pain or oedema, gastrointestinal complaints, or a palpable mass [31] [32]. The classical triad of fever, flank pain, and limitation of hip movement is present in only 30% patients [33,34]. In a majority of cases, iliopsoas abscess occurs secondary to a spinal or extraspinal inflammatory condition, such as spondylodiscitis or Crohn's disease. Primary causes of iliopsoas muscle abscess are rarer, and these arise via haematogenous spread from a focus elsewhere in the body [35].

A small iliopsoas abscess can be treated with broad-spectrum antibiotics; however, collections which are large or unresponsive to medical therapy may require intervention via percutaneous techniques under radiological guidance or open drainage. In one series, patients with bacteraemia who had a small abscess (<3.5 cm) responded well to antibiotics; however, patients with large, complex, or loculated abscesses would likely require drainage [31]. From a series of 41 patients with iliopsoas abscess, it is suggested that collections less than 3 cm in greatest diameter can be managed with antibiotics alone (see Figure 8) [36].

## 5.5 Spinal Immobilisation

A spinal brace, collar, or orthotic device can immobilise the spine to control pain and promote healing by reducing movement.

## 6 Technical Notes and Surgical Pearls

Indications for surgery include SI that is refractory to medical management, negative or unavailable (if deemed unsafe) closed biopsy, SEA or large collection, acute or progressive neurological deficit (from spinal cord, cauda equina, or nerve root compression), delayed instability (secondary to vertebral body destruction), and deformity [37].

The neurological exam and the duration of neurological deficits guide the decision to offer surgery. In an early series of patients with SEA, the group of patients who did not have paralysis or whose paralysis developed less than

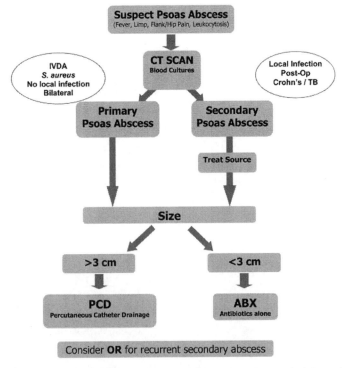

**Figure 8** Algorithm for management of psoas abscess. Copied from (36).

36 hours before their operation had better outcomes compared to the group of patients whose paralysis began greater than 48 hours before surgery. In the latter group, no patient recovered neurological function and all the mortalities were reported in that group [38]. In a series of 87 patients with SEA, it was found that surgical evacuation within 24 hours of MRI identification of SEA versus greater than 24 hours had a relative benefit on discharge neurological status; however, the sample size was too small to reach statistical significance [39]. In a study of 123 patients who underwent early surgery (within 12 hours after admission), delayed surgery (more than 12 hours after admission), or non-surgical management for SEA, better clinical and quality-of-life outcomes were observed in patients undergoing early surgery [40]. Overall, in the context of SEA, the available literature supports that emergency surgical evacuation should be performed as soon as possible once the decision is made to proceed with surgical management, owing to the unpredictable course of SEA and risk of neurological deterioration [41].

Surgical treatment options for SIs (Figure 9) can be classified according to the type of procedure (open versus minimally invasive), approach (anterior, posterior, or combination), and the use of instrumentation [42].

In the cervical spine, an anterior approach (with or without a combined posterior approach) is generally favoured in cases of spondylodiscitis and vertebral osteomyelitis because this provides good access to the vertebral

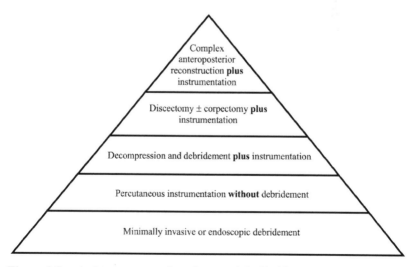

**Figure 9** Surgical treatment options for spondylodiscitis. From bottom to top in increasing complexity and invasiveness. Reference reproduced as a figure from [6]. See CC Rights Link in references.

body and intervertebral disc for debridement and reconstruction (for example, allograft and titanium cage). When corpectomies are required in multiple levels, stability can be achieved with posterior spinal instrumentation and fusion.

In the thoracic spine, anterior approaches include the anterior transthoracic approach, the posterior costotransversectomy, and the extrapleural anterolateral approach. These are utilised for monosegmental, anterior column disease [43]. Posterior laminectomy alone may suffice when SEA is present without anterior column involvement. A combined approach is indicated when there is severe, multi-level anterior column destruction resulting in kyphosis or extensive anterior and posterior column disease. In the thoracic spine, innate stability is afforded by the ribcage so surgical instrumented fusion is not necessarily required, especially if the patient can tolerate an external orthosis [43].

In the lumbar spine, a posterior spinal approach, including laminectomy, can be used to drain a dorsal SEA. However, in cases of discitis and vertebral osteomyelitis, the disease process mainly involves the anterior spinal column. This can lead to delayed instability and a posterior spinal fusion can be performed at the time of the initial operation or in a staged manner.

Use of an excessive amount of foreign material to achieve spinal stability is controversial due to the risk of the foreign material promoting the growth of microorganisms and complicating their eradication. However, the available literature supports the efficacy and safety of internal fixation in SI. Furthermore, implants do not impact healing so long as sufficient debridement has been achieved and the patient receives appropriate antibiotic therapy [44]. Minimally invasive techniques are more technically challenging, but properly selected cases in experienced hands can yield good outcomes.

The choice of surgical technique should be tailored to the expected consistency of the SI, based on the clinic-radiologic findings. When a liquid abscess is expected, then a more minimally invasive technique by way of a laminotomy or hemilaminectomy and irrigation can be used. The patient can be positioned in the reverse Trendelenburg position, utilising gravity to drain liquid abscess. However, when solid granulation tissue is present, then a more extensive, multi-level decompression with focused laminectomies is warranted, assisted by catheter irrigation [6].

## 6.1 Emergency Procedures

### 6.1.1 Posterior Approach for Lumbar Epidural Abscess with/without Discitis

The patient is positioned prone with or without a Wilson frame. A level check is performed, following which the skin and fascia are incised. Muscle is stripped off the spinous processes and laminae. Laminectomy or laminotomy is performed using a drill or rongeurs. If the SEA is liquid, then it can be evacuated with suction and a catheter can be advanced ventrally, as well as cranially and caudally to remove as much pus as possible. However, chronic SEAs may form more solid granulation tissue, or pus that is adherent and mixed with granuloma, which requires use of a combination of pituitary rongeurs and dissectors with suction. The extent of debridement and decompression may necessitate instrumented fusion.

### 6.1.2 Anterior Approach for Cervical Discitis

The patient is positioned supine and a level check is performed. A transverse skin incision is made. The fascia is incised and the platysma is split. The sternocleidomastoid muscle and carotid sheath are retracted laterally. The strap muscles are retracted medially. The pre-tracheal fascia is incised. The longus coli muscles and anterior longitudinal ligament are split and, using subperiosteal dissection, the anterior vertebral body surface is reached.

In cases of spondylodiscitis, this approach permits open debridement of the infected disc. Interbody fusion can be achieved with autogenous or allogenous bone graft. However, extensive vertebral body disease may require corpectomy so a combined posterior approach with instrumentation for stability should be considered as well.

A ventrally located SEA can be drained after dissecting the posterior longitudinal ligament; however, a dorsally located SEA may require a posterior approach.

## 6.2 Relevant Guidelines

Infectious Diseases Society of America (IDSA) Clinical Practice Guidelines for the Diagnosis and Treatment of Native Vertebral Osteomyelitis in Adults [45].

# References

1. Eck JC, Kim CW, Currier BL, Eismont FJ. Infections of the spine. In Steven R. Garfin, Frank J. Eismont, Gordon R. Bell, Christopher M. Bono, Jeffrey S. Fischgrund The Spine. Philadelphia Elsevier; 2018. p. 1256.

2. Enthoven WTM, Geuze J, Scheele J, et al. Prevalence and 'red flags' regarding specified causes of back pain in older adults presenting in general practice. Phys Ther. 1 March 2016;96(3):305–12.

3. Jarvik JG, Deyo RA. Diagnostic evaluation of low back pain with emphasis on imaging. Ann Intern Med. October 2002;137(7):586–97.

4. Premkumar A, Godfrey W, Gottschalk MB, Boden SD. Red flags for low back pain are not always really red: A prospective evaluation of the clinical utility of commonly used screening questions for low back pain. JBJS. 7 March 2018;100(5):368.

5. Grammatico L, Baron S, Rusch E, et al. Epidemiology of vertebral osteomyelitis (VO) in France: Analysis of hospital-discharge data 2002–2003. Epidemiol Infect. May 2008;136(5):653–60.

6. Lener S, Hartmann S, Barbagallo GMV, et al. Management of spinal infection: A review of the literature. Acta Neurochir (Wien). March 2018;160(3):487–96.

7. Mylona E, Samarkos M, Kakalou E, Fanourgiakis P, Skoutelis A. Pyogenic vertebral osteomyelitis: A systematic review of clinical characteristics. Semin Arthritis Rheum. 1 August 2009;39(1):10–17.

8. Stüer C, Stoffel M, Hecker J, Ringel F, Meyer B. A staged treatment algorithm for spinal infections. J Neurol Surg Part Cent Eur Neurosurg. March 2013;74(2):87–95.

9. Corrah TW, Enoch DA, Aliyu SH, Lever AM. Bacteraemia and subsequent vertebral osteomyelitis: A retrospective review of 125 patients. QJM Int J Med. 1 March 2011;104(3):201–7.

10. Murray MR, Schroeder GD, Hsu WK. Granulomatous vertebral osteomyelitis: An update. JAAOS – J Am Acad Orthop Surg. September 2015; 23(9):529.

11. Wiley AM, Trueta J. The vascular anatomy of the spine and its relationship to pyogenic vertebral osteomyelitis. Bone Jt J. November 1959;41B(4): 796–809.

12. Cornett CA, Vincent SA, Crow J, Hewlett A. Bacterial spine infections in adults: Evaluation and management. JAAOS – J Am Acad Orthop Surg. January 2016;24(1):11–18.

13. Calderone RR, Larsen JM. Overview and classification of spinal infections. Orthop Clin North Am. January 1996;27(1):1–8.

14. James SLJ, Davies AM. Imaging of infectious spinal disorders in children and adults. Eur J Radiol. 1 April 2006;58(1):27–40.

15. Silber JS, Anderson DG, Vaccaro AR, Anderson PA, McCormick P. Management of postprocedural discitis. Spine J. 1 July 2002;2(4): 279–87.

16. Bos EME, Haumann J, de Quelerij M, et al. Haematoma and abscess after neuraxial anaesthesia: A review of 647 cases. Br J Anaesth. April 2018;120(4): 693–704.

17. Hong SH, Choi JY, Lee JW, et al. MR imaging assessment of the spine: Infection or an imitation? Radiographics. 2009;29(2):599–612.

18. Tsantes AG, Papadopoulos DV, Vrioni G, et al. Spinal infections: An update. Microorganisms. 27 March 2020;8(4):476.

19. Veljanoski D, Tonna I, Barlas R, et al. Spinal infections in the north-east of Scotland: A retrospective analysis. Ann R Coll Surg Engl [Internet]. 29 July 2022 [cited 6 September 2022]; https://publishing.rcseng.ac.uk/doi/10.1308/rcsann.2022.0062

20. Torrie P, Leonidou A, Harding I, et al. Admission inflammatory markers and isolation of a causative organism in patients with spontaneous spinal infection. Ann R Coll Surg Engl. November 2013;95(8):604–8.

21. Chenoweth C, Bassin B, Mack M, et al. Vertebral osteomyelitis, discitis, and spinal epidural abscess in adults. Guidel Inpatient Clin Care Mich Sch Med. December 2018;

22. Sundaram V, Doshi A. Infections of the spine: A review of clinical and imaging findings. Appl Radiol. August 2016;45(8):10–20.

23. Salaffi F, Ceccarelli L, Carotti M, et al. Differentiation between infectious spondylodiscitis versus inflammatory or degenerative spinal changes: How can magnetic resonance imaging help the clinician? Radiol Med (Torino). April 2021;126(6):843–59.

24. Boudabbous S, Paulin EN, Delattre BMA, Hamard M, Vargas MI. Spinal disorders mimicking infection. Insights Imaging. 4 December 2021; 12(1):176.

25. Marschall J, Bhavan KP, Olsen MA, et al. The impact of prebiopsy antibiotics on pathogen recovery in hematogenous vertebral osteomyelitis. Clin Infect Dis. April 2011;52(7):867–72.

26. Greenberg MS. Destructive lesions of the spine. In Mark S. Greenberg Handbook of Neurosurgery. Ninth New edition. New York: Thieme Medical; 2019. p. 1471–2.

27. Roversi M, Mirra G, Musolino A, et al. Spondylodiscitis in children: A retrospective study and comparison with non-vertebral osteomyelitis. Front Pediatr [Internet]. 2021 [cited 11 September 2022];9. www.frontiersin.org/articles/10.3389/fped.2021.727031

28. Chandrasenan J, Klezl Z, Bommireddy R, Calthorpe D. Spondylodiscitis in children. J Bone Joint Surg Br. August 2011;93-B(8):1122–5.

29. Dayer R, Alzahrani MM, Saran N, et al. Spinal infections in children. Bone Jt J. April 2018;100-B(4):542–8.

30. Bartolo DCC, Ebbs SR, Cooper MJ. Psoas abscess in Bristol: A 10-year review. Int J Colorectal Dis. 1 June 1987;2(2):72–6.

31. Tabrizian P, Nguyen SQ, Greenstein A, Rajhbeharrysingh U, Divino CM. Management and treatment of iliopsoas abscess. Arch Surg. 1 October 2009;144(10):946–9.

32. Shields D, Robinson P, Crowley TP. Iliopsoas abscess – A review and update on the literature. Int J Surg. 1 January 2012;10(9):466–9.

33. Mynter H. Acute psoitis. Buffalo Med Surg J. 1881;21:202–10.

34. Chern CH, Hu SC, Kao WF, et al. Psoas abscess: Making an early diagnosis in the ED. Am J Emerg Med. 1 January 1997;15(1):83–8.

35. Mallick IH, Thoufeeq MH, Rajendran TP. Iliopsoas abscesses. Postgraduate Medical Journal. August 2004;80(946):459–62.

36. Yacoub WN, Sohn HJ, Chan S, et al. Psoas abscess rarely requires surgical intervention. Am J Surg. 1 August 2008;196(2):223–7.

37. Devlin VJ, Steinmann JC. Chapter 67 – Spinal infections. In Devlin VJ, editor. Spine Secrets Plus (Second Edition) [Internet]. Saint Louis: Mosby; 2012 [cited 28 September 2023]. p. 466–72. www.sciencedirect.com/science/article/pii/B9780323069526000762

38. Heusner AP. Nontuberculous spinal epidural infections. N Engl J Med. 1948 Dec 2;239(23):845–54.

39. Ghobrial GM, Beygi S, Viereck MJ, et al. Timing in the surgical evacuation of spinal epidural abscesses. Neurosurg Focus. 1 August 2014; 37(2):E1.

40. Behmanesh B, Gessler F, Quick-Weller J, et al. Early versus delayed surgery for spinal epidural abscess: Clinical outcome and health-related quality of life. J Korean Neurosurg Soc. November 2020;63(6): 757–66.

41. Tuchman A, Pham M, Hsieh PC. The indications and timing for operative management of spinal epidural abscess: Literature review and treatment algorithm. Neurosurg Focus. August 2014;37(2):E8.

42. Guerado E, Cerván AM. Surgical treatment of spondylodiscitis: An update. International Orthopaedics. February 2012;36(2):413–20.

43. Falavigna A, Santos de Moraes OJ. Treatment of discitis and epidural abscess. In Winn. H.R Youmans and Winn Neurological Surgery. Philadelphia. Elsevier. Seventh edition. 2017. 2390–2397.

44. Fontes RBV. Treatment of pyogenic spondylodiscitis. In Youmans and Winn Neurological Surgery [Internet]. [cited 29 September 2023]. pp.

2531–2536.e1. www.clinicalkey.com/#!/content/book/3-s2.0-B9780323 661928003232

45. Berbari EF, Kanj SS, Kowalski TJ, et al. 2015 infectious diseases society of America (IDSA) clinical practice guidelines for the diagnosis and treatment of native vertebral osteomyelitis in adultsa. Clin Infect Dis. 15 September 2015;61(6):e26–46.

Cambridge Elements $^{\equiv}$

# Emergency Neurosurgery

## Nihal Gurusinghe
*Lancashire Teaching Hospital NHS Trust*

Professor Nihal Gurusinghe is a Consultant Neurosurgeon at the Lancashire Teaching Hospitals NHS Trust. He is on the Executive Council of the Society of British Neurological Surgeons as the Lead for NICE (National Institute for Health and Care Excellence) guidelines relating to neurosurgical practice. He is also an examiner for the UK and International FRCS examinations in Neurosurgery.

## Peter Hutchinson
*University of Cambridge, Society of British Neurological Surgeons and Royal College of Surgeons of England*

Peter Hutchinson BSc MBBS FFSEM FRCS(SN) PhD FMedSci is Professor of Neurosurgery and Head of the Division of Academic Neurosurgery at the University of Cambridge, and Honorary Consultant Neurosurgeon at Addenbrooke's Hospital. He is Director of Clinical Research at the Royal College of Surgeons of England and Meetings Secretary of the Society of British Neurological Surgeons.

## Ioannis Fouyas
*Royal College of Surgeons of Edinburgh*

Ioannis Fouyas is a Consultant Neurosurgeon in Edinburgh. His clinical interests focus on the treatment of complex cerebrovascular and skull base pathologies. His academic endeavours concentrate in the field of cerebrovascular pathophysiology. His passion is technical surgical training, fulfilled in collaboration with the Royal College of Surgeons of Edinburgh. Finally, he pursues Undergraduate Neuroscience teaching, with a particular focus on functional Neuroanatomy.

## Naomi Slator
*North Bristol NHS Trust*

Naomi Slator FRCS (SN) is a Consultant Spinal Neurosurgeon based at North Bristol NHS Trust. She has a specialist interest in Complex Spine alongside Cranial and Spinal Trauma. She completed her neurosurgical training in Birmingham and a six-month Fellowship in CSF and Trauma (2019). She then went on to complete her Spinal Fellowship in Leeds (2020) before moving to the southwest to take up her consultant post.

## Ian Kamaly-Asl
*Royal Manchester Children's Hospital*

Ian Kamaly-Asl is a full time paediatric neurosurgeon and Honorary Chair at Royal Manchester Children's Hospital. He trained in North Western Deanery with fellowships at Boston Children's Hospital and Sick Kids in Toronto. Ian is a member of council of The Royal College of Surgeons of England and The SBNS where he is lead for mentoring and tackling oppressive behaviours.

## Peter Whitfield

*University Hospitals Plymouth NHS Trust*

Professor Peter Whitfield is a Consultant Neurosurgeon at the South West Neurosurgical Centre, University Hospitals Plymouth NHS Trust. His clinical interests include vascular neurosurgery, neuro oncology and trauma. He has held many roles in postgraduate neurosurgical education and is President of the Society of British Neurological Surgeons. Peter has published widely, and is passionate about education, training and the promotion of clinical research.

---

## About the Series

Elements in Emergency Neurosurgery is intended for trainees and practitioners in Neurosurgery and Emergency Medicine as well as allied specialties all over the world. Authored by international experts, this series provides core knowledge, common clinical pathways and recommendations on the management of acute conditions of the brain and spine.

Cambridge Elements ≡

# Emergency Neurosurgery

Printed in the United States
by Baker & Taylor Publisher Services